Your No-Nonsense Guide to Crushing Your PA School Interview

By

Francis Sicari, PA-C

Contents

Chapter 1
Congratulations! Let's Get Ready to Crush the Interview!

Kudos, you made it! Congrats on completing the arduous journey to being selected for a PA (physician assistant/physician associate) school interview! You have already accomplished a lot. For many, though, the interview is actually one of the most intimidating and most difficult parts of the PA application process. What will they ask? How many people will be interviewing you? What are they looking for?

I'm here to help. This book is a no-nonsense, BS-proof guide to crushing your PA school interview. A former business consult turned PA, I'm going to hold your hand through the entire process: what they will ask, how you should prepare, what you should wear.

I have to be honest—I always looked forward to interviews, because I felt I was prepared and ready to crush them. In a former life, when I was interviewing for consulting jobs at Ernst & Young, Deloitte, and PwC, I took significant time preparing for interviews. I read books, I took an interview prep course at Penn State, and I practiced my butt off.

Now, I want to share my knowledge and experiences with you so you can crush your PA school interview. So sit back and get ready for this quick-hit guide to crushing your PA interview.

Chapter 2
Dress the Part

It's impossible to overstate the importance of this point. It's often said that up to 90% of communication is non-verbal. I believe it might be even higher, considering factors such as your attire, manner of speaking, and self-assurance. You're not trying to become a hostess at a local bar or the head athletic trainer at a high school, so you don't want to be too casual. Likewise, you're not aiming to be a banker at Goldman Sachs, so a three-piece suit might be overdoing it. You're on the path to becoming a PA—a highly competitive and respected field in medicine. Dress in a way that reflects the prestige of a medical professional.

An important takeaway here is the role of confidence. It's essential to feel confident not just in your preparation, but also in your appearance and demeanor. Typically, it doesn't matter if another candidate in the interview comes from an Ivy League school with a perfect science GPA. Your goal is to present yourself in the best possible light, looking and feeling even more prepared and professional. Confidence is, indeed, key.

This isn't the be-all and end-all, but in my experience these basics will get you by.

What to Wear to Your PA School Interview

For All Applicants

The key to dressing for your PA school interview is to aim for professional and polished attire that conveys respect for the institution and for yourself. You want to ensure that your appearance is neat and that your clothing choices do not distract from the substance of your interview.

For Men

A well-fitted suit in a neutral color such as navy, gray, or black is a classic and safe choice. Pair it with a sharp, coordinating tie and clean, polished dress shoes. Facial hair should be well-groomed, whether you choose a clean-shaven look or a neatly trimmed beard. Your hair should be styled neatly—consider using a small amount of gel if it helps maintain your look. Overall, your outfit should be comfortable enough to allow you to focus on the interview, rather than adjusting your clothing.

For Women

A business professional look is recommended, which can include a tailored pantsuit or a skirt suit in a subdued color. It's best to choose attire that fits well and allows you to sit and walk comfortably. Nails should be manicured in a subtle way; a nude or clear polish will ensure they are presentable without drawing undue attention. Your hair should be styled in a way that it stays out of your face, whether you prefer it curled, straightened, or pulled back. The aim is for a refined look that speaks to your professionalism.

What to Bring

It's not just about dressing the part; it's about showcasing your readiness to engage with the interviewers. Arrive with a professional padfolio that includes paper for notes, along with a good pen. Inside, carry fresh copies of your resume, detailing your experience and academic achievements, as well as your transcripts. Presenting a copy of your resume printed on high-quality paper to your interviewer(s) immediately demonstrates your professionalism and attention to detail. You can find suitable paper at office supply stores like Staples.

Bringing these items not only shows that you're organized and proactive, but also gives you a resource to reference during the interview. It's a subtle yet effective way to set a tone that you're serious and business-oriented about your pursuit of a career as a physician assistant.

General Tips

- Ensure your clothing is wrinkle-free and your shoes are in good condition.

- Keep jewelry and accessories to a minimum; they should not be overly distracting.

- Aim for a natural makeup look, avoiding anything too bold or dramatic.

- It's essential to feel confident and comfortable in what you're wearing, as this will come through in your demeanor.

Remember, the goal of your interview attire is to make a positive, professional impression that complements your qualifications and readiness to become a physician assistant.

Sicari Secret

Navy blue is my go-to color. It's sharp, professional, and will stand out in a group of bland black suits. Complement it with brown shoes and brown leather belt. To complete the look, I always liked to have my padfolio match the brown shoes.

After a few years in consulting, I've learned an undeniable truth: You've got to dress the part. The way you present yourself says a lot about how seriously you take yourself and your aspirations. And I can't overemphasize the importance of feeling good. The last thing you want is to be rummaging through your closet on the day of the interview for a clean button-up or the right pair of shoes. To minimize stress, get everything—your outfit, shoes, the works—dry cleaned and set aside at least a week in advance: Fresh clothes for a fresh you. Let's kick off this process on the right foot.

Chapter 3
Crush the Competition

One aspect often overlooked in other guides is the competitive nature of interview day. Allow me to share some insider information: Interview day is, unequivocally, a high-stress event. For many, this stress can amplify their competitive instincts, particularly among your peers.

It's crucial not to be intimidated by anyone or anything. You might hear boastful claims—someone says they've already been interviewed here, or they've been accepted into a more prestigious school. Perhaps they've conducted research at Harvard or participated in vaccine distribution in Africa.

While commendable, it's important to remember that such remarks are often exaggerated or simply tactics designed to unsettle you. Your focus should be on maintaining a friendly and polite demeanor without engaging in unnecessary competition with the person sitting next to you. Remember, today is about showcasing *your* strengths, not theirs.

Moreover, while you may feel compelled to impress your fellow candidates, keep in mind that they are not the ones evaluating you. I've navigated these waters myself, and I can assure you your goal is to secure your position in PA school with confidence and poise. Direct your energy towards the individuals who hold sway over your admissions decision—the interviewers. Your attention should be laser-focused on this objective.

Sicari Secret

You are going to be stressed! Deep breaths. I like to practice some basic relaxation techniques when I'm stressed. One I like is the 4-5-6 breathing technique. You can do this subtly without anyone noticing. Utilize it when you're waiting for your turn to be called. You are a Zen warrior about to crush it!

Exhale completely*: Begin by letting all the air out through your mouth, making a whooshing sound.*

Inhale for 4 seconds*: Close your mouth and quietly inhale through your nose to a mental count of 4.*

Hold for 5 seconds*: Hold your breath for a count of 5.*

Exhale for 6 seconds*: Exhale completely through your mouth for a count of 6.*

Keep it cool and collected. Here's the inside scoop—everyone around you in that interview waiting room is likely just as jittery. You're there decked out in your best, totally focused, ready to dazzle. I've been in the trenches of consulting interviews, where it often felt like an elaborate display of one-upmanship. It's a similar vibe at PA school interviews, like everyone's silently vying to outdo the last.

But here's a golden nugget of advice: Save that competitive energy. Your real audience isn't the other applicants; it's the interview panel. You're there to make a genuine connection with them, not to compete in an unspoken contest of credentials with your peers.

Redirect all that intensity into your interactions with the interviewers. Let your enthusiasm for the PA profession show, and infuse your responses with the genuine passion you feel. It's your personal narrative and authentic engagement that will make you memorable, not just the sheen of your shoes or the GPA you earned.

Keep that energy reserved for those who are there to find the bright new stars of the program—and let that be you.

Sicari Secret

Do not over caffeinate! Do you normally drink caffeine? If so, be sure to have your normal cup of coffee. But if you don't normally drink caffeine or think you need extra, don't do it. Last thing you want on interview day is anxiety and jitters.

Chapter 4
Introduction and Elevator Pitch

Imagine this scenario: You're seated, your heart racing as you wait your turn. Then, suddenly, it's your moment—your name is called. "Frank, are you ready to come in?" This is your opportunity, and thanks to countless rehearsals and my guidance, you're fully prepared.

As you enter the room, you're greeted by one or several individuals—typically two or three. While your appearance is already professional, it's now crucial to embody professionalism fully. You confidently approach each person, offering a handshake and introducing yourself, "Hello, I'm Frank, pleasure to meet you!" Remember, a firm handshake, steady eye contact, and unwavering confidence are your keys to making a stellar first impression.

Now seated, the interview officially begins. Often, and almost always, it will start with a prompt along the lines of, "So, Frank, tell me about yourself." This is what I refer to as your elevator pitch—a term I didn't invent, but one that is pivotal. This brief introduction, lasting about 30 seconds, is your chance to convey who you are and what you stand for. It's a critical moment that shapes the entire interview. The concept of an elevator pitch is named for its brevity, like the duration of an elevator ride, where you concisely share a key point or two and establish a connection. Although you're not in an actual elevator, the principle remains the same.

In the upcoming sections, I'm going to guide you through creating your perfect elevator pitch, step by step. With around 30 interviews under my belt spanning consulting, PA school, and various job hunts, I can tell you this: The "Tell me about yourself" prompt is almost inevitable. I want you to be so well-prepared for this moment that when your interviewers ask it, your eyes light up like a batter at the sight of the perfect pitch. Let's knock this one out of the park together.

You want to craft your statement to highlight your passion for the medical field, relevant experiences, and personal attributes that make you a strong candidate for PA school, while adding a personal touch. Here's how you can structure it.

Planning Your Elevator Pitch

Introduction and Academic Background

Start with a brief introduction of yourself, including your educational background and any relevant healthcare experience.

_____

_____

_____

_____

_____

_____

Professional Experience and Healthcare Exposure

Clearly articulate why you want to become a physician assistant. Mention what specifically draws you to this field and how your past experiences have led you to this decision.

_____

_____

_____

_____

_____

_____

Personal Qualities and Career Aspirations

Discuss any clinical experience, volunteer work, or educational background that has prepared you for PA school. Highlight specific skills or experiences that align with the role of a PA, such as teamwork, patient care, or problem-solving abilities.

_____

_____

_____

_____

_____

_____

Career Goals

Briefly mention your long-term career aspirations within the PA profession.

_____

_____

_____

_____

_____

_____

Call to Action and Connection With the Program

Conclude by expressing your strong interest in the program and your eagerness to contribute to and learn from it.

_____

_____

_____

_____

_____

Elevator Pitch Planning: My Example

Having trouble getting started? Check out my responses below.

Introduction and Academic Background

"Hello, I'm a proud graduate of Pennsylvania State University, where I embarked on an exciting journey blending my interests in healthcare and business. After earning my degree, I ventured into healthcare consulting with PwC, one of the world's leading consulting firms. My passion for medicine didn't stop there; I pursued further academic enrichment through a post-baccalaureate program at Stony Brook University, excelling in rigorous science courses. This unique blend of experiences has laid a solid foundation for my future in healthcare."

Professional Experience and Healthcare Exposure

"My journey toward becoming a physician assistant is deeply rooted in my lifelong passion for medicine and a hands-on, active lifestyle. Working in healthcare consulting provided me with a broad perspective on the industry, but it was my direct experiences shadowing in an emergency room and scribing in urgent care that solidified my decision. These roles allowed me to witness the critical impact of PAs firsthand, fueling my desire to be part of a team that makes a tangible difference in patients' lives on a daily basis."

Personal Qualities and Career Aspirations

"My background in the fast-paced world of consulting, combined with clinical experience, has equipped me with essential skills for a PA, such as effective communication, empathy, and the ability to thrive under pressure. I am hardworking, personable, and deeply passionate about healthcare. These qualities, paired with my clinical experiences, make me well-suited for the dynamic and challenging role of a physician assistant."

Career Goals

"Looking ahead, I am eager to specialize in emergency medicine. The fast-paced environment of the ER is where I feel most energized and where I've seen the invaluable role of PAs in providing critical care. I aspire to be part of that bustling environment, making swift decisions that save lives and contribute significantly to patient care."

Call to Action and Connection to the Program

"I am particularly drawn to Summit View for its reputation as a top PA program in the area. Having heard firsthand accounts from alumni who are now thriving in medicine, I am confident Summit View is where I can further my aspirations. I am excited about the opportunity to contribute to and learn from a program that values excellence and innovation in healthcare."

Engagement Question

"As I prepare for the challenges and rewards of PA school, I would love to know more about how Summit View supports its students in navigating the rigorous curriculum and clinical rotations. Are there specific resources or programs in place that have been particularly beneficial for students?"

General Tips for a Successful Pitch

- **Conciseness and coherence**: Keep your message brief and focused, ensuring it flows smoothly from one point to the next without rushing through important details.

- **Passion and confidence**: Deliver your pitch with genuine enthusiasm and belief in your ability to succeed in the PA program and your future career.

- **Practice**: Rehearse your pitch to ensure it sounds natural and you can deliver it confidently.

Remember, the goal of your pitch is not just to list your qualifications, but to tell a compelling story about why you are drawn to the PA profession and how your background has prepared you for this career path.

My Elevator Pitch

Now let's put it all together. Here's my elevator pitch, which highlights my educational background, relevant experiences, motivation for becoming a PA, and my interest in the specific program. It's concise, yet comprehensive, and ends with an engaging question that demonstrates my interest in the program. Remember, practicing your pitch will help you deliver it more confidently and naturally.

"Thank you for this opportunity to interview. I'm Frank Sicari, a Penn State graduate with a passion for medicine. I enhanced my academic foundation at Stony Brook University with rigorous science courses.

"My role in healthcare consulting at PwC, along with shadowing in an emergency room and scribing in urgent care, solidified my commitment to patient care. I'm hardworking, personable, and aim to thrive in an emergency room setting.

"I'm excited about the Summit View PA program due to its stellar reputation and the success of its graduates. To better prepare myself, could you share what qualities and experiences your program values most in a candidate?"

Sicari Secret

We'll delve into this more deeply later, but it's crucial from the outset not to express a desire to work in a specialized field, such as dermatology or cosmetics, during your interviews. Highlighting such interests can be off-putting to interviewers, who are primarily looking for candidates eager to serve in broader, more generalist roles such as primary care and emergency medicine— areas where PAs are most needed. Recall the origins of this profession: It emerged in response to a doctor shortage during wartime. The last thing interviewers want to hear is that your primary goal in attending PA school is to specialize in aesthetic procedures like Botox and fillers. Instead, they are looking for future PAs who are ready to embrace the challenges of primary care and emergency medicine, helping to narrow the gap between scarce healthcare resources and the high demand for these essential services. This commitment to general care is, after all, the foundation upon which the PA profession was built.

You know why I'm all about nailing that elevator pitch, right? It's your golden ticket to making a splash with that very first question. Ace it, and you'll not only boost your own confidence sky-high, but you'll also signal to the interviewers that you've got your act together. First impressions? They're huge. So, craft a killer elevator pitch and then drill it to perfection. I'm talking about practicing so much that you could do it in your sleep—that's the level we're aiming for.

Now It's Your Turn!

Write your elevator pitch here.

_____

_____

_____

Chapter 5
The Basics of the Profession and Your Program

Before we delve into the nuanced behavioral and situational questions that are integral to your PA program interview, it's essential to first grasp the fundamentals of the PA profession and the specifics of the program you're considering. It's crucial for you to be comfortable with the basics: understanding the origins and objectives of the PA profession, and how the role of a PA differs from that of other healthcare providers.

This knowledge is not just academic; it's likely to form the basis of interview questions about your decision to pursue a career as a PA. Remember, your choice to become a PA wasn't arbitrary; it was a well-researched decision, informed by a thorough understanding of the alternatives. Similarly, when it comes to the specific program you're applying to, being armed with key facts and details can significantly bolster your interview performance. Let's start with a concise overview of these essential points.

The PA Profession

Basics and History of the Physician Assistant Profession

The physician assistant (PA) profession has its roots in the mid-20th century in the United States, born out of a necessity to address a growing healthcare challenge.

Origins of the Profession

The inception of the PA profession dates back to the mid-1960s, a period marked by a critical shortage of primary care physicians. This deficit was especially pronounced in rural and underserved areas, paving the way for the creation of the PA role to help alleviate this issue.

Dr. Eugene Stead's Vision

A key figure in the establishment of the PA profession was Dr. Eugene A. Stead, Jr. from Duke University Medical Center. Drawing inspiration from the rapid and efficient training of doctors during World War II and the proficiency of medical corpsmen, Dr. Stead founded the first PA program. This pioneering program welcomed its inaugural class in 1965 at Duke University.

The Role's Evolution

Following Duke University's lead, other institutions began to introduce PA programs, signaling the early adoption and institutional support for this emerging profession. Initially focused on primary care, the scope of the PA role has since broadened significantly to include a wide range of medical specialties.

Impact on Healthcare

PAs have played a pivotal role in bridging the healthcare gap, significantly enhancing the accessibility of medical care, particularly in areas previously underserved by doctors. As the demands of healthcare have shifted and expanded over the years, the role of PAs has evolved accordingly, cementing them as an indispensable part of the healthcare delivery system.

Comparing Education and Scope of Practice

Physician Assistants (PAs)

PAs obtain a master's degree from an accredited program, typically taking about two years, followed by 2,000 hours of clinical rotations after classroom and lab instruction in medical sciences. Compared to doctors, PAs follow a shorter and more cost-effective educational path, allowing for quicker entry into the healthcare field. They enjoy greater career flexibility, being able to switch specialties without additional formal education.

Limitations of a PA

The scope of practice for PAs includes diagnosis and treatment, often under the supervision of a physician, although their level of autonomy can vary by state. They are authorized to prescribe medications in most states, provided they have the necessary DEA registration. PAs can specialize across various fields, albeit with some procedural limitations, and typically consult with physicians on more complex cases. The ability to prescribe controlled substances is also granted, subject to state regulations and DEA registration requirements.

Medical Doctors

Their educational journey includes a bachelor's degree, four years of medical school, and 3–7 years of residency training. Doctors undergo extensive education in medical sciences and gain prolonged clinical experience. This pathway is longer and more expensive compared to that of PAs.

Nurses

Nurses may earn a bachelor's degree in nursing (BSN), an associate degree, or a nursing diploma, focusing their clinical training on patient care, community health, and long-term care. Compared to PAs, nurses have a more limited scope of practice, with PAs able to diagnose, treat, and prescribe medications across various medical specialties.

Nurse Practitioners (NPs)

NPs advance their education with degrees such as MSN (Master of Science in Nursing) or DNP (Doctor of Nursing Practice) following registered nurse (RN) certification. Their clinical training ranges from 500–1,000 hours in specific health areas. While NPs also have a significant degree of autonomy and can specialize, PAs have the edge in terms of the ease with which they can change specialties. PA training, which is akin to medical school, provides versatility that allows them to work in diverse roles, including surgery and emergency medicine, areas that might be less accessible for NPs.

Knowing Your PA Program

As you prepare for your PA school interview, it's vital that you thoroughly understand the key aspects of the program you're considering. This insight is not just about assessing whether the program aligns with your own needs and goals; it's also about your ability to clearly express during the interview why you are interested in the program and how you're a great fit for it. Let's explore the best ways for you to approach and understand these crucial elements.

Understanding and Leveraging Key Program Aspects

- **Class size:** Understand whether the program has a larger or smaller class size. Smaller classes can provide personalized attention and stronger peer interactions, while larger ones may offer diverse perspectives and more networking opportunities.

- **Articulate your fit**: In the interview, explain how the class size suits your learning style. For instance, if you prefer intimate learning environments, highlight how a smaller class size supports your educational success.

- **Attrition rate as an indicator of program stability**: Investigate the program's attrition rate. A lower rate typically indicates student satisfaction and a supportive educational environment. If the rate is low, emphasize how this reassures you about the program's stability. If it's high, inquire about strategies in place to support student success.

- **PANCE first-time pass rate as a measure of preparation**: The Physician Assistant National Certifying Examination (PANCE) pass rate reflects the program's effectiveness in preparing students. A high rate suggests efficient teaching and comprehensive preparation. You can comment on how a high pass rate boosts your confidence in the program's ability to equip you for a successful PA career.

- **Accreditation a non-negotiable criterion**: Verify that the program is accredited by the ARC-PA or a similar body. Accreditation is vital for PANCE eligibility. Convey awareness and demonstrate your understanding of accreditation's importance in your career trajectory and its influence on your program choice.

- **Staff-to-student ratio**: A favorable staff-to-student ratio usually translates to better faculty access and a more personalized educational experience. Highlight its importance to a quality education. Discuss how the staff-to-student ratio will enhance your learning experience and your appreciation for close mentorship and guidance.

By understanding these aspects and incorporating them into your interview responses, you demonstrate not only your thorough research about the program, but also your proactive approach to ensuring it's the right fit for your educational and professional aspirations. This level of preparedness and insight can be impressive to interview panels and may help set you apart as a candidate.

Chapter 6
A Framework for Answering Any Question: The STARR Method

Like anything else you're doing and want to do well, it's important to have a framework for your interview strategy. While attending Penn State's business school, I took a professional development course where in addition polishing our professional skills, we also focused heavily on interviewing. The method I learned there has been invaluable tool to crushing interviews, and I'm going to share it and review it with you here. It's called the STARR Method.

The STARR Method for answering interview questions, particularly behavioral and ethical/scenario-based questions, will provide a structured and effective approach. The STARR Method is an adaptation of the commonly known STAR (Situation, Task, Action, Result) method, with an added element of Reflection, which is crucial in healthcare professions like PA. Here's a more detailed breakdown:

- **Situation**: Set the stage by describing the context or scenario vividly.

- **Task**: Define the specific challenge or problem you were tasked with addressing.

- **Action**: Detail the specific steps and actions you took to resolve the challenge.

- **Result**: Share the outcomes and results of your actions.

- **Reflection**: Conclude by reflecting on the lessons learned from the situation, whether positive or negative, highlighting your ability to grow and learn from experiences. This aspect is particularly crucial for demonstrating your self-awareness and capacity for improvement during interviews.

This framework provides you with a logical guideline for narrating a story and emphasizing the main point. The scenario could unfold as follows. The interviewer asks you a question: "Can you tell me about a stressful time during one of your experiences in healthcare and how you dealt with it?"

Let's use the STARR method to breakdown this question.

Question: Can you tell me about a stressful time during one of your experiences in healthcare and how you dealt with it?

- **Situation**: Begin by vividly describing the situation you were in. Paint a picture for your interviewer. *During my clinical role in an urgent care facility, a patient became increasingly upset due to a long wait time, making a scene and agitating other patients and staff.*

- **Task**: Explain the task or problem you needed to address. *As the doctors and PAs were occupied with other patients, it fell upon me to intervene and calm the agitated patient while diffusing the situation.*

- **Action**: Detail the specific actions you took to accomplish the task. *I approached the patient calmly, extending my apologies and empathizing with their frustration. I explained the emergent situation that had caused the delay and assured them that we would attend to them as soon as possible. To ease their discomfort, I offered a cold bottle of water, which they gratefully accepted.*

- **Result**: Describe the outcome of your actions. *The patient gradually calmed down, allowing us to prioritize their care. After the consultation, the patient not only apologized for their outburst but also expressed gratitude for our understanding and assistance.*

- **Reflection**: Conclude by reflecting on what this experience taught you and whether you gained insights, positive or negative. *This situation reinforced the importance of compassion and empathy in healthcare. It taught me that even in challenging circumstances, there is always an opportunity to connect with difficult patients when approached with understanding. Additionally, I learned the value of quick thinking and effective communication during moments of tension.*

As you can see, the STARR method provides a structured approach for dissecting a question, allowing you to craft your response logically and effectively. It serves as a versatile framework for tackling various interview questions.

Let's explore another example, this time an ethical question that doesn't come with a specific task or situation embedded in it. Can the STARR method still be applied? Absolutely.

Question: What would you do if, as a PA, you didn't agree with your supervising physician's approach to a patient?

- **Introduction**: This question presents a common ethical dilemma often faced by PAs in the field. Here's how I've navigated such situations in the past.

- **Situation**: During my time at a physical therapy office, we had a young female patient recovering from an ACL injury, but her progress was slower than expected. Her major obstacle was an inability to tolerate the pain resulting from the required manual manipulation to break up scar tissue. The physical therapist I was assisting wanted me to hold her down against her will during this painful procedure.

- **Task**: I found myself in a difficult position, as I wasn't comfortable with the situation. However, my supervisor insisted this was the only way to advance her recovery. My discomfort was particularly heightened as the patient was a 14-year-old girl in significant pain.

- **Action**: I mustered the courage to express my concerns to the physical therapist, making it clear that I was uncomfortable participating in this manner. The following day, I took the matter up with the head PT, and we engaged in a dialogue about the situation. Together, we explored alternative approaches to enhance the patient's treatment outcomes.

- **Result**: The head of the physical therapy clinic convened a meeting with the patient's physical therapist and the patient's parents to discuss the treatment plan and its progression. Ultimately, it was collectively agreed that physically restraining the patient was not a suitable long-term strategy.

Instead, the patient was referred back to the orthopedist for additional assessments to ensure proper healing.

- **Reflection**: My core values drive me to uphold ethical medical practices, even in the face of disagreement with superiors. I am committed to ensuring the well-being of the patient and will not compromise on that principle. As a PA, I would apply this same value system, always striving to do what's right and bringing concerns to the attention of superiors and managers when necessary.

Consider Possible Scenarios

Is the STARR method suitable for every interview question? While it isn't a universal solution, it undoubtedly provides a strong foundation for addressing a wide range of questions. Consider that interviewers typically have a limited timeframe, usually just 30 to 60 minutes, to assess your qualifications.

Given this time constraint, here's a strategic suggestion: Focus your preparation on outlining 10 scenarios using the STARR method. These scenarios should encompass diverse experiences from the past five to 10 years, drawn from your professional background or personal life, as each offers valuable insights.

Your time might be better spent delving deeply into a few situations that you're comfortable reflecting on, rather than attempting to cover a hundred potential questions. The key is to feel at ease with your responses; your answers to interview questions should flow naturally. By immersing yourself in a select set of experiences, you'll be better equipped to discuss them comfortably, resulting in a more compelling presentation on your part.

In the upcoming chapter, we're about to jump headfirst into some targeted questions. But hold your horses! Before we do that, I've got a lineup of 15 scenarios for you to mull over. Picture this as your personal patchwork of experiences, stitched together to give you that confident edge when you're in the hot seat for PA school interviews.

Here's your mission: Sift through these scenarios and link each one to a story or experience from your own life. Think of it as loading your bow with arrows, each one an anecdote ready to be fired off when the moment strikes. No need to craft full answers now—just match them up. Ready to get those wheels turning and spark some storytelling flair? Let's make it happen!

Example Scenarios

Communication: Share instances where you've effectively utilized your communication skills in challenging situations.

_____

_____

_____

_____

_____

_____

Family stressor/trauma: Reflect on a personal tragedy you've faced and how you navigated through it.

_____

_____

_____

_____

_____

_____

Conflict resolution: Describe scenarios where you successfully resolved disputes, whether among team members, colleagues, or in personal contexts. Highlight the steps you took to achieve positive resolutions.

_____

_____

_____

_____

_____

_____

Stress management: Discuss your approach to handling stressful situations effectively.

_____

_____

_____

_____

_____

Ethical dilemmas: Narrate experiences involving ethical dilemmas and your responses to them.

_____

_____

_____

_____

_____

Teamwork: Share times when you've worked effectively as part of a team, detailing your contributions and the outcomes achieved.

_____

_____

_____

_____

_____

Specific healthcare situation: Discuss impactful healthcare-related experiences you've been part of.

_____

_____

_____

_____

_____

_____

Leadership experience: Detail instances where you assumed leadership roles, outlining challenges faced and how you led teams to success.

_____

_____

_____

_____

_____

_____

Adaptability: Describe situations where you adapted to significant changes or overcame unexpected challenges.

_____

_____

_____

_____

_____

_____

Patient advocacy: If applicable, talk about instances where you advocated for patient needs or rights, even when facing obstacles or resistance. Highlight the impact of your advocacy on patient care.

_____

_____

_____

_____

_____

_____

Time management: Share scenarios where you effectively managed multiple tasks or responsibilities within tight deadlines.

_____

_____

_____

_____

_____

_____

Continuous learning: Reflect on experiences that demanded rapid acquisition of new knowledge or skills, detailing your learning approach and practical applications.

_____

_____

_____

_____

_____

_____

Crisis management: Narrate situations where you played a role in managing crises, whether medical emergencies, workplace crises, or other critical circumstances.

_____

_____

_____

_____

_____

_____

Patient education: If applicable, discuss experiences where you educated patients or their families on complex medical conditions or treatment plans. Describe how you ensured understanding and compliance.

_____

_____

_____

_____

_____

_____

Quality improvement: Talk about scenarios where you identified opportunities for quality improvement in your work or organization, explaining the steps taken to address issues and the positive outcomes achieved.

_____

_____

_____

_____

_____

_____

By immersing yourself in these scenarios in advance, you'll be exceptionally well prepared to respond confidently and effectively to a wide spectrum of interview questions, ultimately showcasing your adaptability and readiness for PA school interviews.

Chapter 7
Navigating the Tough Questions: A Strategic Approach

When it boils down to it, interviewers tend to focus on just a handful of key topics—they just have different ways of approaching them. My aim here isn't to hand you the perfect response to every question, but to equip you with a solid foundation so you can confidently tackle a variety of questions. I'll also provide potential responses as examples to get your creative juices flowing.

Remember, your answers shouldn't necessarily mirror mine, but having an example can kickstart your thought process. Where applicable, let's aim to apply the STARR method we discussed earlier. Now, let's take a high-level look at the basic question categories before diving into each one in detail.

Question Categories

Motivational Questions

- Why do you want to become a physician assistant?

- What inspired you to pursue a career in healthcare?

- What makes the PA profession appealing to you compared to other healthcare roles?

Educational and Experience-Based Questions

- Tell us about your academic background and how it has prepared you for PA school.

- Describe any healthcare-related experiences you have, such as volunteering, shadowing, or working in healthcare settings.

- What challenges have you faced in your education or healthcare experiences, and how did you overcome them?

Ethical and Scenario-Based Questions

- How would you handle a situation where a patient refuses treatment?

- Describe a time when you faced an ethical dilemma, either in your personal life or during your healthcare experience. How did you resolve it?

- Can you discuss a current issue in healthcare and how it might impact the role of PAs?

Behavioral Questions

- Give an example of a time when you had to work under pressure. How did you manage it?

- Describe a situation where you had to work as part of a team. What was your role, and what was the outcome?

- Can you tell us about a time when you had to demonstrate empathy or compassion?

Personal Attribute Questions

- How would you describe your strengths and weaknesses?

- What qualities do you believe are essential for a successful PA, and how do you embody these?

- How do you handle stress, and what do you do to maintain a healthy work–life balance?

Goal-Oriented Questions

- Where do you see yourself in five to 10 years after completing PA school?

- What are your career goals, and how does becoming a PA fit into these goals?

- What specialties in medicine are you interested in, and why?

Program-Specific Questions

- Why have you chosen to apply to our PA program?

- How do you plan to contribute to our program and the PA community here?

Questions About Current Healthcare Issues

- What are some of the biggest challenges facing healthcare today?

- How do you think the role of PAs will evolve in the coming years?

- Can you discuss a recent advancement in healthcare and its implications for PAs?

Applying the STARR Method

Let's break this down together. I'll take each question, and where the STARR method— Situation, Task, Action, Result, and Reflection—fits, we'll plug it in. Along the way, I'll drop some pointers to keep things spicy. Now, my responses aren't the gold standard, and mimicking them isn't the game plan. They're more like a springboard for your own memories. Hopefully, you'll catch glimpses of your own experiences in mine and get a feel for how I weave them into my answers.

Also, pay attention to the conversational tone in my replies. You're human, and your answers should be as well—ditch the script! Aim for a chatty, relaxed tone. If you rehearse without becoming a parrot, you'll come off as genuine and smooth when it counts. Let's make your prep so spot-on that when interview day rolls around, you'll be chatting like you're with old friends!

Motivational Questions

Question: Why do you want to become a physician assistant?

Question breakdown: This question might seem straightforward, especially after dedicating the last 4–8 years of your life to securing this interview spot. However, articulating your passion for medicine can sometimes be challenging. Let's take a measured approach to ensure you convey your motivations clearly and effectively.

Inspiration could come from various sources. Was it a significant event in your life, such as a family member's illness, or perhaps shadowing a PA, that sparked your interest in joining the ranks? Being a PA offers many tangible benefits, including excellent compensation, a flexible work schedule, the ability to move between specialties, direct involvement in surgeries, and a lesser burden of debt compared to medical school.

An ideal answer might start with a heartfelt sentiment but also touch upon the practical benefits toward the end.

My response: "Why do I want to become a PA? My interest in medicine and healthcare has always been strong, but it wasn't until I had the opportunity to shadow a PA in the emergency room that I was truly captivated by the profession. Observing the PA handle a diverse range of patients and conditions—not just performing procedures like suturing, prescribing medication, and starting IVs, but also playing a key role in coordinating the emergency room by communicating effectively with nurses and doctors—was incredibly inspiring. The job's daily challenges and its impactful role in healthcare, combined with my research into the growing need for PAs, the field's expansion, and the economic advantages over medical school, solidified my decision to pursue this path. I am as excited now about entering this field as I was the day I first shadowed a PA in the ER."

Alternative points: It's important to avoid mentioning motivations that could be perceived negatively. Statements such as "I couldn't get into medical school," "I didn't want to be a nurse," or "I want to be a cosmetic injector" should be kept to yourself. Even if these factors played a part in your decision, focus on the positive aspects of becoming a PA. Your interviewers are looking for candidates who are passionate about the role and understand the PA's crucial position in healthcare—serving as a bridge to underserved communities, filling gaps in care, and being on the frontlines of patient treatment.

* * *

Question: What inspired you to pursue a career in healthcare?

Question breakdown: This question is like the one above, and it's perfectly acceptable during an interview to refer back to your previous answers. You might say, "As I mentioned earlier, my shadowing experience in the ER significantly solidified my interest in healthcare." However, let's provide more context about who you are to your interviewers.

My response: "During my undergraduate years at Penn State, I was deeply involved in the school's dance marathon, an annual fundraiser aimed at fighting pediatric cancer. Organizations on campus would fundraise and spend time with the affected families throughout the year. The sense of fulfillment from participating in this cause was indescribable. In my final year, I was chosen to represent my fraternity in the grueling 48-hour dance marathon, which involved no sitting or sleeping. The event raised millions in donations and was one of the most rewarding experiences of my life. There has been nothing else in my life that has given me as much satisfaction as helping others. I realized then that I wanted to continue making a difference in people's lives, and this profession offers the perfect opportunity to do so."

Sicari Secret

It's perfectly acceptable to showcase your achievements during these interviews. Prepare to highlight your accomplishments, but do so with subtlety. If you've reached this stage, you undoubtedly have notable achievements worth mentioning. The key is to brag modestly. For instance, referencing my involvement in the dance marathon often led to more detailed discussions about my time at Penn State and the event itself. Discussing your experiences in depth not only showcases your achievements but also strategically reduces the time available for additional questions. So, come prepared with your achievements, ready to share them in a manner that naturally complements the conversation.

Alternative points: It's important to avoid discussing financial incentives, such as knowing a PA who earns a significant income from performing cosmetic procedures. Likewise, the desire to wear a white coat for the sake of professionalism should not be a driving factor. We are healthcare providers, not stockbrokers; our motivation should reflect our commitment to care and service.

Additional considerations: If you have a sick family member who received exceptional care, a mentor or colleague who inspired you, or family members in healthcare (for example, "My mother was a nurse, and my sister is a healthcare professional. I come from a family of caregivers; it's in my blood."), these are valuable points to mention. Sharing such personal stories can highlight your inherent passion for healthcare and underscore the values that drive you towards this profession.

* * *

Question: What makes the PA profession appealing to you compared to other healthcare roles?

Question breakdown: I recommend beginning with your passion for being a PA and the day-to-day realities of the role. However, I would only delve into the key differences between MDs, NPs, and PAs if specifically asked in the question.

My response: "The medical field offers many remarkable paths, such as becoming an MD, nurse practitioner, or physical therapist. However, what captivated me about the PA profession was witnessing PAs in action. Observing their daily activities, skills, and the leadership roles they embrace within the healthcare system truly made an impact on me. My experience wasn't limited to shadowing a PA in the emergency room just once; I did it for several months. I also spent time shadowing a PA in the ICU and gained insight into other healthcare roles through my family, with both my mother and my sister working as nurses. Additionally, I completed some of my clinical hours in a physical therapy office, working closely with physical therapists. Despite this broad exposure, the PA profession stood out to me. Its focus on leadership, the opportunity to perform a variety of procedures, and the ability to engage in hands-on patient care highlighted it as the most compelling way for me to make a significant difference."

When discussing why not an MD or NP, if prompted, I'd highlight the *pragmatic* aspects—like the PA's flexibility, the focused yet comprehensive medical education without the staggering debt associated with medical school, and the medical model training that differs from the nursing model. These elements, along with the PA's versatility across specialties and the presence in emergency settings, align closely with my aspirations and areas of interest.

Response expanded: "The PA profession encapsulates the best of all worlds. It allows me to pursue a lifelong passion for medicine in a financially and practically viable manner. Becoming a PA enables me to fulfill a dream in the most balanced way possible."

Alternative points: It's crucial to steer clear of motivations such as financial gain, fallback options (such as not getting into medical school), or targeting niche roles as primary reasons. The focus should remain on the broader appeal of the PA profession and its unique contributions to healthcare.

Educational and Experience-Based Questions

Question: Tell us about your academic background and how it has prepared you for PA school.

Question breakdown: Let's be clear, you and your fellow interviewees will come from similar backgrounds, but there are opportunities to distinguish yourself from the crowd. Indeed, everyone has taken rigorous science courses and likely boasts a high cumulative GPA, but what other challenges have you faced? Did you work full-time or part-time? Were you an athlete or involved in time-consuming extracurricular activities? Interviewers are looking to see if you can manage a heavy workload. How did you balance academic responsibilities with other life commitments? Furthermore, do you consider yourself a lifelong learner? Discuss your ongoing education beyond just the mandatory coursework. What unique aspects of your experiences set you apart?

My response: "My academic journey is somewhat unique. I started off at Penn State's business school, focusing on healthcare, and then worked in PwC's healthcare consulting division for two years. I gained a number of insights from the corporate world, but my real passion lay in medicine, leading me to pursue a post-baccalaureate pre-health program at Stony Brook. Known for its rigorous science courses, Stony Brook challenged me but I thrived, earning a 3.9 GPA. During this time, I also worked full-time as a medical scribe in urgent care and shadowed PAs in both the ER and ICU. These experiences not only honed my ability to manage multiple responsibilities simultaneously—a skill I believe is essential for PA school—but also reinforced my commitment to healthcare. I'm a lifelong learner, always eager to engage with classroom work and apply it to real-world scenarios."

Alternative points: While discussing your academic and professional background, it's important to remember that a high GPA, while impressive, is not the sole focus. Keep in mind, all candidates at this stage have likely excelled academically. The admissions panel is keen to assess your commitment to the PA program and ensure there's minimal risk of you not completing the course. Steer clear of mentioning personal circumstances that could be perceived as potential distractions, such as a long-distance relationship, plans to work alongside your studies, or time-consuming hobbies. Instead, emphasize your readiness and wholehearted commitment to the PA program, demonstrating that you are fully prepared and dedicated to this path.

* * *

Question: Describe any healthcare-related experiences you have, such as volunteering, shadowing, or working in healthcare settings.

Question breakdown: This question can come in different forms, but essentially, it's about what lights that fire within you. Did you simply tick off boxes, or were you genuinely excited about your work? Even if not every day was a highlight in your clinical role, try to recall and share those moments or cases that truly energized you. Reflect on whether your experience was limited or if you had a broad spectrum of experiences to draw from.

My response: "I've been really lucky to have had some genuinely thrilling experiences in healthcare so far. I've shadowed two PAs in areas I'm particularly drawn to, the ER and ICU. I also worked in a physical therapy office, gaining insights into orthopedic injuries and rehabilitation processes. However, my most cherished and extensive experience was as a medical scribe in urgent care.

Sure, there were stressful days, but I genuinely enjoyed every day I spent there. The fast pace, the range of cases we saw, and the variety of diagnoses we worked up were incredibly educational. That role didn't just teach me a lot; it cemented my determination to pursue this career path."

Alternative points: If your experiences in healthcare are on the limited side, don't let it worry you. Remember, quantity doesn't always mean quality. Focus on giving depth to any experiences you do share, and convey your genuine enthusiasm for the work you were involved in. It doesn't matter whether you were performing chest compressions in the ER or providing basic care in a nursing home; the interviewers are looking for candidates who have witnessed the less glamorous sides of healthcare but still possess an unwavering passion and commitment to advancing in the field.

* * *

Question: What challenges have you faced in your education or healthcare experiences, and how did you overcome them?

Question breakdown: This question might feel familiar, kind of like when someone asks "What's your biggest weakness?" or "Tell us about a time you failed." The trick here is to demonstrate that you're the kind of person who learns from their mistakes, doesn't make the same mistake twice, and has the ability to adapt and grow when unexpected challenges pop up.

So, let's use the STARR method to tackle this question effectively.

- **Situation**: During my post-baccalaureate program at Stony Brook, I tore my ACL playing basketball. For someone as active as I am, who relies on physical activity to manage stress, it hit hard.

- **Task**: Initially, I struggled with the injury and the sudden halt to my active lifestyle, not to mention the logistical nightmares it caused on a campus as spread out as Stony Brook's. Juggling a demanding course load with my new physical limitations was tough, but I didn't let it stop me.

- **Action**: Instead, I found a silver lining by picking up a new hobby: playing the guitar. What started as a makeshift stress relief became a passion—I got quite good at it, and it's now a regular part of my life, offering both mental engagement and relaxation.

- **Result**: This experience didn't just teach me a new skill; it gave me a deeper appreciation for my health and resilience. Nowadays, I continue to lead an active lifestyle, focusing on gym workouts and running, albeit more mindfully and with an emphasis on less strenuous activities.

- **Reflection**: Through this experience, I learned the importance of adaptability and finding alternate paths to achieve my goals. It reinforced my belief in the power of positivity and resilience in overcoming challenges.

Now let's put it together.

My response: "During my post-baccalaureate program at Stony Brook, I tore my ACL playing basketball. For someone as active as I am, who relies on physical activity to manage stress, it hit hard. Initially, I struggled with the injury and the sudden halt to my active lifestyle, not to mention the logistical nightmares it caused on a campus as spread out as Stony Brook's. Juggling a demanding course load with my new physical limitations was tough, but I didn't let it stop me. Instead, I found a silver lining by picking up a new hobby: playing the guitar. What started as a makeshift stress relief became a passion—I got quite good at it, and it's now a regular part of my life, offering both mental engagement and relaxation. This experience didn't just teach me a new skill; it gave me a deeper appreciation for my health and resilience. Nowadays, I continue to lead an active lifestyle, focusing on gym workouts and running, albeit more mindfully and with an emphasis on less strenuous activities."

Alternative points: It's best not to discuss experiences such as failing a course, putting social life before academics, or showing an inability to learn and evolve from challenges. The goal is to highlight resilience and growth, not to dwell on setbacks without demonstrating positive outcomes.

Ethical and Scenario-Based Questions

Question: How would you handle a situation where a patient refuses treatment?

Question breakdown: Encountering a patient who refuses treatment is a scenario you're likely to face during your PA career. It could stem from various reasons, whether religious beliefs or disagreements with the proposed treatment plan by a family member. Regardless of the specifics, as a healthcare provider, your role remains consistent: to educate, offer options, and strive for better outcomes. In reality, these situations are not uncommon, and interviewers want to see how you approach them with a level-headed demeanor. There's no one-size-fits-all solution; instead, they're interested in observing your logical navigation through ethical dilemmas.

Applying the STARR method:

- **Situation**: During my time shadowing healthcare professionals, I've witnessed numerous instances where patients or their family members declined treatment or testing, especially during the peak of the pandemic.

- **Task**: Despite presenting troubling symptoms, some patients refused COVID testing or transfer to the hospital, emphasizing the challenge of respecting patient autonomy while ensuring their well-being.

- **Action**: While I didn't take direct action, these experiences emphasized the importance of not imposing care on anyone. Instead, I learned that our role as medical professionals is to provide information and present options to empower patients in decision-making.

- **Result**: Through these experiences, I reinforced the significance of patient education, highlighting the risks associated with non-compliance in a clear, non-confrontational manner.

- **Reflection**: This turbulent period underscored the multifaceted responsibilities we'll face as healthcare providers. Beyond diagnosis and treatment, effective communication with patients, even amidst disagreement, is vital for providing optimal care.

My response: "In my time shadowing healthcare professionals, I've witnessed several instances where a patient or their family member refused treatment or testing. During the peak of the pandemic, for instance, numerous patients either outright refused COVID testing or declined transfer to the hospital despite presenting troubling vitals. What these experiences have taught me is that our primary duty is to educate patients and their families, presenting them with options. Ultimately, the decision rests with the patient and their loved ones on how to proceed with the information and options provided. Our responsibility is to ensure they have access to the best possible information and choices to foster positive outcomes."

Alternative points: Steer clear of implying any sort of coercion or manipulation when it comes to treatment decisions; it's all about being honest and maintaining integrity when sharing information. Adding personal stories really brings your answer to life. Have you ever faced ethical dilemmas like this during your shadowing or clinical experiences? Sharing these firsthand experiences not only deepens your understanding, but also highlights your skill in handling complex situations ethically and with empathy.

* * *

Question: Can you discuss a current issue in healthcare and how it might impact the role of PAs?

Question breakdown: Think of this question as a golden opportunity handed to you on a silver platter! PAs are in the perfect position to tackle myriad current challenges in healthcare. From the dearth of primary care providers to the shortage of healthcare workers, not to mention the issues of escalating costs and declining outcomes, PAs stand out as a key part of the solution. In your response, I want you to highlight this vital role of PAs. Focus on the positive impact and avoid framing any issue as a setback for PAs. This question is your chance to show that you understand and embrace the broader vision of what PAs can achieve in the healthcare system.

My response: "A pressing issue in healthcare today is the scarcity of primary care, largely due to a shortage of doctors. Primary care physicians are often seen as the 'quarterbacks' of a patient's healthcare team, and the lack of accessible primary care could lead to suboptimal health outcomes. Specialists have their vital roles, but now more than ever it's crucial for patients to undergo annual physical exams and complete their preventive care screenings. Our aim is to prevent health issues before they arise and provide treatment when necessary. Fortunately, this is where our profession—physician assistants, along with other advanced practice providers—plays a critical role. We are poised to bridge these gaps, and I believe we will significantly contribute to enhancing patient outcomes and overall care quality."

Alternative points: Try not to delve into controversial topics—notice how I approached the answer by identifying a challenge but also highlighting a positive aspect. This approach can be applied to any sensitive topic. For example, when discussing opioids, you could mention that many patients turn to these drugs due to a lack of access to appropriate care, framing the discussion in a way that acknowledges the problem while also suggesting constructive ways to address it.

Behavioral Questions

Question: Give an example of a time when you had to work under pressure. How did you manage it?

Question breakdown: Let's face it, healthcare is incredibly rewarding but doesn't come without its share of stress. And guess what? PA school is no walk in the park either. Your interviewers are on the lookout for candidates who've been through the wringer and come out stronger. So, let's dig deep into your experiences and pull out a time when you not only faced a challenge head-on but learned something invaluable in the process. Remember the STARR method we talked about? This is the perfect moment to put it into action. The interviewer wants a concrete example. By applying the STARR method, you'll do more than just recount the situation; you'll analyze and reflect on it, showing them that you've faced stress, managed it like a pro, and even thought about ways you could've handled things even better.

Applying the STARR method:

- **Situation:** During my final semester at Stony Brook University, I faced my heaviest course load yet while juggling two jobs and applying to PA school.

- **Task**: My goal was to excel academically, maintain work responsibilities, and fulfill all requirements for PA school applications.

- **Action**: To manage the pressure, I decided to buckle down and prioritize my commitments. I reduced gym visits from five days to two and a half and cut back on social engagements. Though challenging, I saw these sacrifices as temporary and necessary for long-term goals.

- **Result**: Despite the demands, I had one of my most successful semesters. I maintained a high science GPA, completed all CASPA requirements, and secured several PA school interviews while meeting work obligations.

- **Reflection**: This period taught me to focus on priorities and manage time effectively. I realized temporary sacrifices are often crucial for long-term success. It bolstered my confidence in handling pressure and highlighted the importance of balancing personal and professional commitments to avoid burnout.

My response: "During my final semester at Stony Brook University, I faced immense pressure. Juggling a heavy course load, two jobs, and PA school applications demanded effective time management and prioritization. I decided to cut back on non-essential activities like gym sessions and socializing, recognizing these sacrifices as necessary for achieving my goals. Despite the challenges, I emerged from this period with one of my most successful semesters. Maintaining a high GPA, completing all application requirements, and securing PA school interviews validated the effectiveness of my approach. Reflecting on this experience, I realized the importance of focus and temporary sacrifices for long-term success. It instilled in me the confidence to handle pressure and reinforced the significance of balancing personal and professional commitments to prevent burnout."

Alternative points: When discussing personal sacrifices, emphasize their role in achieving goals rather than portraying them negatively. Personal reflections enhance your response, showcasing self-awareness and growth potential.

* * *

Question: Describe a situation where you had to work as part of a team. What was your role, and what was the outcome?

Question breakdown: Here's another opportunity to showcase your teamwork skills, and I see these kinds of questions as softballs. You can choose any situation, whether it's from your clinical experiences, shadowing, or academic life. It's important to show the interviewers that you're a well-rounded individual, so don't feel restricted to only using healthcare experiences. When I was interviewing, I liked to include aspects of my involvement in sports and my fraternity. Let's apply the STARR method, and I'll review my response.

Applying the STARR method:

- **Situation:** I was elected as the homecoming chair for my fraternity.

- **Task**: My responsibilities included coordinating with visiting alumni, collaborating with our paired sorority to plan social events and build a float for the parade, and ensuring our fraternity house was in top shape for the alumni's arrival.

- **Action**: I delegated tasks to various fraternity brothers, assigning one to oversee the float, another to assist in organizing social events with the sorority, and a third to liaise with the alumni. Meanwhile, I acted as the central point of contact and coordinator for all activities.

- **Result**: The weekend's events were a resounding success, with a fantastic turnout and positive feedback from both brothers and alumni. It was a rewarding experience that showcased our teamwork and leadership abilities.

- **Reflection**: While it was undoubtedly a stressful week, I found immense satisfaction in overcoming challenges and seeing the successful outcome. This experience taught me valuable lessons about effective delegation, communication, and teamwork.

My response: "I've been fortunate to participate in numerous team settings, particularly in sports and healthcare, but one experience stands out as particularly challenging yet rewarding. I was elected as the homecoming chair for my fraternity, tasked with coordinating a week of events, communicating with alumni, organizing social activities with our paired sorority, and constructing a float for the parade. It was a demanding role, but I leveraged the strengths of my fraternity brothers by delegating specific responsibilities. Despite the workload, the weekend was a tremendous success, and it taught me invaluable lessons about collaboration and leadership. This experience truly prepared me for future challenges where teamwork is essential."

Alternative points: Emphasize how the experience challenged you and helped you grow. Highlight specific skills or lessons learned from the teamwork experience.

* * *

Question: Can you tell us about a time when you had to demonstrate empathy or compassion?

Question breakdown: When we talk about healthcare, compassion isn't just a nice-to-have, it's a cornerstone of the care we provide. Let's delve into a time when I had the chance to put compassion into action—preferably during a healthcare experience. This is a perfect moment to apply the STARR method, so let's break it down.

- **Situation**: My colleague and I are wrapping up for the day. Unexpectedly, we hit a snag—our patient is without a ride home. My colleague is in a bind, needing to leave immediately for a family matter that simply can't wait.

- **Task**: Even though I had mentally checked out for the day, I wasn't about to leave our patient in a bind. The task in front of me was straightforward but important: ensure that this patient, already facing a challenging day, isn't abandoned.

- **Action**: I stepped up. I reassured my colleague that family commitments should always come first and insisted she attend to her matters. Meanwhile, I stayed back, keeping our doors open a tad longer, and struck up a friendly conversation with the patient while we waited for his ride.

- **Result**: It was a 20-minute wait for the cab, but eventually, it arrived. As he left, the patient expressed his gratitude with a simple "thank you" that resonated with a depth of meaning that went beyond words.

- **Reflection**: Looking back, I was completely spent—both physically and emotionally drained. But there was this undeniable glow of contentment. It's experiences like this that truly underline the "care" in healthcare. It's not just about addressing the physical ailments; it's about touching and healing the human spirit, sometimes just by being there.

My response: "You know, there's this particular day at the urgent care that's etched in my memory. We were winding down from what had been a relentless 12-hour shift when this gentleman walked in. His appearance was a bit worn—clothes showing a bit of life's wear and tear, his mannerisms somewhat curt—and it was clear as day that he was carrying some heavy mental health struggles. Despite his rough approach and less-than-warm attitude, we provided him with the care he needed, no questions asked.

"As the clinic was about to close, the provider I was working with faced a dilemma. They had urgent commitments that couldn't be postponed, but our patient was still awaiting his ride. In that moment, I decided to volunteer to lock up the clinic and wait with him, to make sure he wouldn't have to linger outside alone.

"Honestly, after such a long day, all I could think about was heading home. But my conscience nudged me to stay. The thought of him, clearly someone with not many advocates in his corner, being left to wait in the dark just didn't sit right with me. When his ride finally showed up—about 20 minutes later—I saw a certain relief in his eyes. His 'thank you' as he left was brief, but it was heavy with gratitude that you don't come across every day.

"It validated my choice to stay back. That 'thank you' wasn't just common courtesy; it was a heartfelt acknowledgment of a simple act of kindness. Heading home, I felt a deep sense of satisfaction, knowing I had lived up to the spirit of healthcare—it's all about compassion, one patient at a time."

Personal Attribute Questions

Question: How would you describe your strengths and weaknesses?

Question breakdown: This question is an invaluable exercise, doubling as a chance to tackle two significant questions that are commonly asked in interviews: pinpointing your paramount strength and admitting a weakness. It's a subtle art; the challenge is to present your strengths with confidence without veering into arrogance, and to discuss your weaknesses without casting doubt on your overall abilities.

Navigating your greatest weakness: When it comes to weaknesses, honesty is crucial. Yet, the real purpose of this question isn't just to reveal a shortcoming. Rather, interviewers are interested in how you recognize and address your weaknesses. The focus should be on your self-awareness, the steps you're actively taking to mitigate your weaknesses, and how you're converting them into opportunities for personal growth. It's not merely about confessing a flaw; it's about showing adaptability and a dedication to continual self-enhancement.

Showcasing your strengths: Conversely, discussing strengths is your opportunity to modestly spotlight what you bring to the table. This is the moment to affirm the positive traits you possess. Whether you're notably sociable, or you have an unwavering work ethic, it's advantageous to offer a concrete example that demonstrates how your strength has been beneficial in a professional setting. The aim is to articulate how this particular trait distinguishes you and adds value to your role or workplace. It's less about the strength itself and more about the impact of that strength on your performance and contributions.

Ultimately, while tackling this question, keep the narrative centered around you as a reflective individual—one who understands their ongoing path of personal and professional growth.

And yes, that STARR framework could even be applied here!

- **Situation**: At the physical therapy office where I worked, there was a piece of equipment, specifically an older model traction machine, that I was initially hesitant to use due to its complexity and infrequency of use.

- **Task**: My task was to overcome my hesitation and unfamiliarity with the traction machine in order to become a more versatile and competent member of the physical therapy team.

- **Action**: I took the initiative to come in on my day off and ask for training from a physical therapist. I dedicated extra time to learning and practicing with the traction machine until I felt confident in my ability to use it effectively.

- **Results**: As a result of my efforts, I transformed my apprehension into proficiency with the traction machine, expanding my skill set and contributing more fully to the team.

- **Reflection**: This experience reinforced the value of stepping out of my comfort zone, and the importance of continuous learning. It showed me that embracing challenges is essential for growth, and this mindset will serve me well in my aspiration to become a physician assistant, where adaptability and the pursuit of knowledge are crucial.

My response: "In assessing my weaknesses, I've realized that staying within my comfort zone was holding me back. I've learned that growth often comes from stepping into the unfamiliar, embracing discomfort as a catalyst for improvement. A prime example of this was my initial hesitation to use the traction machine at the physical therapy office where I worked. It was an older, rarely used model, and I found it quite daunting. I avoided it for a year, until I decided to confront this reluctance. On my day off, I sought out training with a physical therapist and quickly transformed my apprehension into proficiency.

"As for my strengths, they manifest most notably in my robust work ethic and my readiness to seek out growth opportunities. The initiative I took to master the traction machine is just one instance of this. I am proactive, never hesitating to ask for help, to seek additional training, or to invest extra time into mastering new skills. This approach has consistently rewarded me with enhanced abilities and knowledge, which I believe are essential qualities for a physician assistant. I am dedicated to continuous learning and expanding my competencies to provide the best care possible."

Sicari Secret

Whether or not the question is posed in the manner above, it's always advantageous to acknowledge a weakness but pivot to highlight a strength. Reframe the question in such a way that the focus shifts from dwelling on a weakness to emphasizing your ongoing commitment to self-improvement.

Question: What qualities do you believe are essential for a successful PA, and how do you embody these?

Question breakdown: Interviewers seek to understand not only if you recognize the qualities necessary to be a successful physician assistant, but also how you embody these characteristics in your own experiences. It is always beneficial to illustrate your points with specific examples.

Consider discussing the following key qualities, though your exploration should not be limited to these alone:

- Leadership
- Commitment to continuous learning
- Communication skills
- Empathy
- Adaptability
- Problem-solving skills
- Teamwork
- Clinical competence

- Resilience under stress

My response: "My perspective is that being a physician assistant is a multifaceted role that demands an individual with a diverse skill set and a well-rounded character. In my view, the key qualities essential for a successful PA include adaptability, a commitment to continuous learning, and clinical competence. These attributes not only distinguish PAs but are also traits that I possess and have consistently demonstrated.

"My adaptability has been proven through my experience in diverse professional environments. I have not only thrived in the corporate sector within a top-tier firm, but have also excelled academically in Stony Brook's post-baccalaureate pre-health program, known for its rigorous science courses.

"Moreover, my passion for learning is ever present. I am an enthusiastic reader, always keen to acquire new skills or insights. This is particularly important in the healthcare field, where medicine is continuously advancing. I understand the imperative of keeping abreast of these changes, which directly ties into the value of lifelong learning.

"Lastly, my varied background, having worked with different populations and in various healthcare roles, has given me a broad base of knowledge and the versatility to flourish in multiple settings. My experiences range from the corporate sector to a physical therapy office and an urgent care clinic. This diversity in my professional journey is what sets me apart, making me a polished and well-rounded candidate. I am eager to leverage my skills and experiences to excel in the PA role."

* * *

Question: How do you handle stress, and what do you do to maintain a healthy work–life balance?

Question breakdown: We've touched on this before: Medicine can be a pressure cooker. It's not just about experiencing stress—it's about showing that you've got a grip on it. Can you stay cool when the heat is on, or does the pressure get to you? It's alright to draw from all walks of life here—athletics, academics, and especially those make-or-break moments in healthcare.

The STARR method breakdown:

- **Situation**: One day at the urgent care we were two scribes short, and the waiting room was overflowing. The providers were under tremendous pressure to see patients quickly without compromising the quality of care.

- **Task**: My role was to ensure accurate and efficient documentation of medical records, allowing the providers to focus on patient care without additional administrative burdens.

- **Action**: I prioritized my workflow, focusing on the most critical cases first, and communicated closely with the medical team to stay ahead of the curve. I also utilized shorthand techniques that I had developed over time to speed up the process without sacrificing detail.

- **Result**: Thanks to these strategies, we managed to get through the day without significant delays in care. Patient records were up to date, and the providers could maintain their focus on treatment.

- **Reflection**: This experience underscored the value of staying calm under pressure. Outside of work, regular exercise is my go-to stress reliever, keeping me physically and mentally agile. Moreover, I make sure to carve out time for activities that rejuvenate my spirit, like hiking and reading. This balance enables me to return to each shift with a clear head, ready to support the healthcare team and tackle whatever challenges come our way.

My response: "One particularly stressful day when we were understaffed and the clinic was overwhelmed with patients during the height of COVID stands out. The community was hit hard, and every patient needed thorough attention and swift documentation to keep up with the pace of care.

"Even though it was incredibly stressful, I stayed focused and didn't let my attention to detail waver. What I've learned from working in high-stress situations is the importance of not overreacting. The goal remains to work hard and put forth your best effort. To effectively manage this, I've found that maintaining a healthy work–life balance is crucial. After work, I decompress through exercise and spending quality time with friends, which helps me enjoy my downtime and come back to work recharged."

Alternative points: Of course I don't want you saying you cave under pressure. Demonstrate to your interviewers that you have been under stress and can handle it with a clear head. Again, it's okay to reference something outside of a healthcare setting, such as sports.

Goal-Oriented Questions

Question: Where do you see yourself in five to 10 years after completing PA school?

Question breakdown: This question really zooms in on your future vision and understanding of the PA role. For the first five years, it's a good idea to focus on sharpening your skills, possibly in one of the environments we've talked about such as the ER, primary care, or within a hospital setting. And when looking further down the road, mentioning any aspirations to step into administration or take on a teaching role could definitely score you some extra points!

My response: "In the short term, I picture myself caring for patients in an emergency room setting, diving into the thick of it. I'm all about mastering my craft in those first few years, from handling urgent cases to fine-tuning my procedural abilities. Looking further ahead, I see myself stepping into a leadership position. With my business background, I can definitely envision a pivot into an administrative role later on, all while keeping a hand in clinical practice. I believe I have the leadership chops and organizational savvy to really thrive in an admin capacity."

Additional points: Think about incorporating a commitment to continuous education into your vision. Envision yourself possibly mentoring the next generation of PAs as a clinical instructor, which not only demonstrates your dedication to the profession but also emphasizes your leadership potential.

Reflect on how you could engage with the broader community through your role. Showing interest in public health initiatives, policy development, or community outreach can illustrate a holistic approach to your career in medicine.

Don't forget to touch on personal development. Balancing professional aspirations with personal growth can make you stand out as a well-rounded candidate. Convey how maintaining interests outside of medicine can contribute positively to your role as a healthcare provider and help prevent burnout. In framing your answer, aim to present a well-rounded picture that includes not just your career trajectory but also how you plan to contribute to the field and your own self-care.

* * *

Question: What are your goals outside of your professional career, and how does becoming a PA fit into these goals?

Question breakdown: So, we all have career aspirations, right? But what's life without a bit of balance? Maybe you want a family, or perhaps you've got some big dreams outside the nine-to-five. Me? I'm all about finding that sweet spot. Sure, I'm passionate about my work in healthcare, but I'm just as enthusiastic about lacing up for triathlons. It's all about not letting work or life tip the scales too much. This question isn't just about your professional goals; it's about showing you're a well-rounded individual who'll mesh with the student community.

My response: "For the last six years, I've been all in—gathering healthcare experience, acing my courses, and working toward becoming a PA. But there's more to me than that. Triathlons are my passion outside of medicine. I've got this great crew I train with, and each year, we push each other a little harder, go a little faster. While my career takes the lead, I'm also looking forward to furthering my triathlon goals and, hey, starting a family with my fiancée. We're both locals and can't wait to plant our roots even deeper here."

Additional points: PA programs love it when they see you're keen on getting involved locally. They're not just training clinicians; they're cultivating community leaders. It's a big plus if you can show you're excited to serve the areas around the school. Sure, we might end up wherever the wind—or the acceptance letters—takes us, but hinting at a commitment to the local scene can definitely earn you some extra credit.

* * *

Question: What specialties in medicine are you interested in, and why?

Question breakdown: Here's a pitch right in the strike zone—let's hit a homerun! We've gone over this, but it bears repeating: Stating that your ultimate goal is to work in a niche field like dermatology or cosmetic surgery could be a misstep. While those are admirable pursuits, remember that PA programs are often geared towards addressing broader healthcare needs. They're looking for candidates eager to serve in high-demand areas such as primary care, emergency medicine, and hospital medicine. Even if those aren't your top choices, avoid signaling a narrow focus too early on.

My response: "The appeal of the PA profession for me is its incredible flexibility. I've watched friends thrive in fast-paced ERs, intensive care units, and various specialties. Yet, it's the dynamic environment of the emergency room that captivates me. The experience I gained while shadowing ER professionals was exhilarating—the variety of cases and the chance to perform intricate procedures is what drives me."

Additional points: If the conversation turns to specialties, it's fine to acknowledge your openness to exploring different areas while emphasizing that initially you'd like to sharpen your skills in foundational practices, such as primary care or emergency medicine. Remember, it's important to appreciate the value of all fields within medicine, not just the ones that currently pique your interest. Last thing you want to do is downplay a specialty and come to find out your interviewer works in that specialty.

Program-Specific Questions

Question: Why have you chosen to apply to our PA program?

Question breakdown: So, you're suited up and you've hit the books to prep for this interview, but is this really where you want to spend the next few crucial years of your life? I'd bet the answer is a resounding *yes*. Now, it's all about making the interviewers believe that too. If I know someone who's been part of the program or is an alum, I always try to bring that up. Maybe it's a friend who's graduated and can't stop raving about their experience, or someone who's now killing it in the ER, just where I aim to be. And as we've covered earlier, you should be all over the program's key stats like a pro—think low attrition rate, impressive PANCE pass rates, or their ties to a renowned hospital system. Don't forget the more personal factors. Is the campus a stone's throw from your family home? Can you commute and save some cash? These details can be game-changers for your success. Keep it real—sure, any acceptance letter would make your day, but let's make it clear why *this* place feels just right.

My response: "I've dedicated myself fully to this path and would be overjoyed to be accepted into any program. However, your school feels like the perfect fit for me. Being accepted here means I would have the added benefit of living at home, surrounded by a solid support network that I'm confident will help me excel. My friend Noel, an alumna of your program, now excels in her work at Peconic's emergency room and speaks very highly of her experience. What really clinches it for me are the compelling aspects of your program—the impressive low attrition rate, the excellent PANCE pass rates, and the ideal class size."

Alternative points: If they throw you a curveball, asking if you've applied elsewhere, it's totally fine to acknowledge that. It would be unwise not to cast a wide net. But here's the kicker—make it clear from the get-go that while any program acceptance would be great, you believe you'd do your best work right here.

* * *

Question: How do you plan to contribute to our program and the PA community here?

Question breakdown: Are you someone who contributes to the community? Do you work well with others? Will you integrate seamlessly into our program? Interviewers are looking for candidates eager to succeed, but who are also willing to help their peers excel. Consider your ability to collaborate in team settings, maintain a positive attitude through highs and lows, and how you've engaged in academic collaboration in the past. Have you served as a teaching assistant for any classes?

My response: "I believe I would be a valuable addition to your program. I maintain a positive mindset and am quite sociable. I'm excited about the prospect of making friends and creating study groups to collectively understand and succeed. At Stony Brook, I forged strong friendships within my courses, and we collaborated effectively to tackle complex subjects, particularly in organic chemistry. I also served as a teaching assistant for anatomy, which allowed me to help others while solidifying my own knowledge. I plan to continue this collaborative spirit in the program."

Additional points: Emphasize your strong work ethic and dedication to being a team player. Remember, this journey is not a solo competition; it's about learning and thriving together with your classmates.

Questions About Current Healthcare Issues

Question: What are some of the biggest challenges facing healthcare today?

Question breakdown: Healthcare is a complex, ever-evolving puzzle, presenting myriad challenges: soaring costs, suboptimal outcomes, workforce shortages, the opioid crisis, and the looming threat of provider burnout. It's essential to be well-versed in these topics—not only to excel in your interview, but also to prepare yourself for the real-world scenarios you will encounter. A pro tip: When concluding your answer, highlight how PAs are positively impacting the healthcare landscape.

My response: "The mismatch between the high costs of healthcare and the quality and patient outcomes we observe is one of the industry's most pressing issues. It's time we celebrate high-quality care and positive patient experiences. This is where PAs come into the limelight. I recently read an article about a study that illustrated that care provided by PAs is not only cost-effective but also rivals, and sometimes surpasses, the care delivered by MDs. I'm ready to jump in and contribute to the solution, armed with a zeal for medicine and a readiness to make a tangible impact."

Alternative points: Notice how I referenced a recent study? It's an effective way to show that you're engaged with current research and industry trends. It's also wise to navigate clear of politically sensitive topics during an interview. While you may have strong opinions on issues like abortion rights or fluctuating healthcare policies, an interview isn't the venue for debates, given that opinions can vary widely.

* * *

Question: How do you think the role of PAs will evolve in the coming years?

Question breakdown: Now, it's a given that our field is up and coming—and so are the opportunities that come with it. Sure, we could talk about the obvious stuff like PAs getting more independence. But let's not stop there. There's a whole buffet of topics we could serve up, like stepping up in policy-making, zooming in on specialties, or widening our practice playground.

My response: "When it comes to the evolution of PA roles, the prospects are genuinely exhilarating. There's a palpable increase in the need for medical care, which paves the way for PAs to step into roles with more autonomy, especially in hospitals and primary care. But the bigger picture is even more exciting. I see PAs stepping up to the plate in leadership, shaping healthcare policy, and steering the direction of healthcare administration. With our robust training, hands-on clinical experience, and advanced education, we're not just prepared to fill these shoes—we're ready to sprint in them.

"And as for my personal goals? I'm eager to embrace a leadership position, actively contribute to improving community health, and advocate for the growth and development of our profession. It's about harnessing our collective potential to make a lasting impact."

Additional points: Notice how in my response I didn't just offer my thoughts on the future—I wove in my aspirations to contribute to that future. It's a subtle yet powerful way to show interviewers that you're invested in the profession's growth. It echoes the timeless wisdom of JFK: It's not just about what the profession can do for us, it's what we can do for the profession—and for each other as PAs.

Now that we've tackled some the bigger topics and provided a framework for answering these questions, lets jump into some of the curveballs you may encounter interview day.

Chapter 8
Curveballs: Quizzes, Writing Samples, and Strange Questions

Hopefully at this point you have come to realize the interview is not just about nailing every question. You need to dress the part, act the part, and exemplify to the staff at the program that you are the real deal.

Besides the questions we've already chewed over, you might get thrown a curveball or two—like writing samples, pop quizzes, or even questions that come out of left field. Let's pull back the curtain on this part of the interview process so that when the big day rolls around, you won't be caught off guard.

Navigating Quizzes

It might come as a surprise, but yes, some PA school interviews include a short quiz. From my own journey and conversations with peers, it's not uncommon to face a quick-fire round of 10 to 20 questions. These aren't meant to stump you; they're to ensure you've got a solid foundation. Let's make sure you walk in ready to impress.

Here's what you might be up against and what you'll want to have down pat.

- **PA profession's backstory**: It's crucial to understand the history of the physician assistant profession. Find out how the field was established, who the pioneers were, and what key events have defined its progress.

- **Medical terminology 101**: Familiarize yourself with the basic language of medicine. While you don't need to memorize the entire medical dictionary, knowing common terms and phrases is important. If your experience with medical terminology is limited, consider picking up a beginner's guide.

- **Specifics of the program**: Research thoroughly the program for which you are interviewing. Learn about their mission, what they are known for, and tailor your preparation to the particular characteristics that make them stand out.

- **Ethical brain teasers**: Be prepared to tackle ethical dilemmas during your interview. These questions are less about finding correct answers and more about demonstrating your ability to thoughtfully navigate through complex issues.

Remember, the quiz isn't just a test of knowledge—it's a showcase of your preparation and enthusiasm for the PA path. So, take a deep breath, brush up on these areas, and go show them what you're made of!

Submitting a Writing Sample

In addition to the possibility of quizzes, you may also be asked to produce a writing sample. As a PA, it's imperative to have strong writing and communication skills for tasks such as completing SOAP notes and liaising with medical colleagues or insurance companies. I recommend revisiting the foundational principles of composition you would have encountered in English or history classes. Think of it as constructing a document-based question (DBQ): Begin with an introduction that presents your main argument alongside three supporting points, continue with three paragraphs to expand on each point, and conclude with a summary that reinforces your argument.

Here's a concise example for reference.

Assigned Topic

In recent months, there has been significant media coverage on the global effort to combat the resurgence of measles, a disease previously well-controlled by vaccination. This has sparked a widespread debate on public health policy, individual rights, and community responsibilities.

Considering the recent outbreaks, write a brief essay discussing the role physician assistants should play in addressing vaccine hesitancy among patients. How can PAs effectively communicate the importance of vaccinations to prevent such outbreaks, and what strategies could be implemented in clinical practice to increase vaccination rates? Additionally, reflect on how PAs can balance respecting patient autonomy with ensuring public health safety.

Essay Response

Introduction: The resurgence of measles, a disease once on the brink of eradication in many parts of the world, underscores a growing public health concern: vaccine hesitancy. As frontline healthcare providers, physician assistants (PAs) are uniquely positioned to address this challenge. Their accessibility, coupled with the trust they foster in clinical settings, empowers them to play a critical role in public health advocacy and education, particularly regarding vaccinations.

Supporting paragraph 1: Firstly, PAs can leverage their frequent patient interactions to educate individuals about the benefits and safety of vaccines and provide evidence-based information to debunk common myths and misconceptions. By personalizing the conversation and addressing specific concerns, PAs can help patients make informed decisions. This approach requires not only a deep understanding of immunology and public health, but also empathy and communication skills to connect with patients on a personal level.

Supporting paragraph 2: Secondly, PAs can implement strategies in clinical practice to improve vaccination rates. This can include setting up reminder systems, providing walk-in vaccination services, and working with healthcare teams to create a culture of immunization within the practice. By making vaccines more accessible and convenient, and by routinely assessing patients' vaccination status, PAs can significantly increase uptake and contribute to herd immunity in the community.

Supporting paragraph 3: Furthermore, PAs must navigate the delicate balance between respecting patient autonomy and protecting public health. This involves ethical decision making, and sometimes difficult conversations with patients who are reluctant to vaccinate. PAs should advocate for vaccinations not just as a protective measure for the individual patient, but as a social responsibility to safeguard vulnerable populations, such as immunocompromised individuals, who rely on herd immunity for protection against contagious diseases.

Conclusion: In conclusion, the role of physician assistants in combating vaccine hesitancy is multifaceted and indispensable. Through education, practical strategies in clinical settings, and ethical advocacy, PAs have the potential to be influential proponents of vaccinations. Their contributions are vital in bridging the gap between public health directives and individual patient care, ultimately steering communities towards safer and healthier futures. As we face the resurgence of preventable diseases, the proactive efforts of PAs are more important than ever in promoting the well-being of society at large.

Prepare for Possible Writing Sample Topics

You don't need to burn the midnight oil writing a bunch of essays in advance. But, it's a smart move to brush up on the key points we've talked about. Maybe grab a coffee, pull out a notepad, and scribble down your top three takeaways for each topic. Think of it as your interview cheat sheet—it's not about memorizing answers, but having those solid ideas in your back pocket. This way, you can walk into that interview with confidence, ready to knock that essay out of the park.

Here a few other topics you could encounter:

- **Healthcare ethics**: Tackle the ethical dilemmas healthcare professionals encounter, such as end of life decisions, confidentiality breaches, and allocating limited medical resources.

- **Professional challenges**: Explore the potential challenges in the PA profession and strategies for overcoming them.

- **Current healthcare topics**: Discuss recent healthcare legislation, the role of technology in healthcare, and major public health issues such as the opioid epidemic or responses to pandemics.

- **Personal reflection**: Reflect on personal experiences that have equipped you for the PA role, or share your motivations for choosing this career path.

- **Case studies**: Analyze hypothetical patient scenarios, decision making in patient care, and collaboration with the healthcare team.

- **Teamwork and collaboration**: Emphasize the significance of collaborative work in healthcare and your approach to interdisciplinary teamwork.

- **The role of the PA**: Share your insights into the PA's responsibilities within the healthcare system and your anticipated contributions to the field.

- **Healthcare policy**: Offer your viewpoint on policy debates impacting PAs, such as practice scope or access to healthcare.

- **Healthcare disparities**: Address healthcare inequality, barriers to care for marginalized groups, and ways to promote health equity.

- **Patient education and advocacy**: Discuss the PA's duties in educating and advocating for patients, and how you'd communicate with patients about their healthcare.

When preparing for these topics, it's helpful to stay informed about current events in healthcare and to reflect on your personal experiences and beliefs related to the PA profession. Remember, the goal of the writing sample is to demonstrate your ability to think critically and communicate effectively, not necessarily your expertise on the topic itself.

Curveball Questions

Sometimes you will get a question that doesn't seem to have a right answer and, honestly, it may *not* have one. That's okay—the goal isn't to answer the question right per se, but to demonstrate you can handle ambiguity and work through it logically.

Let's quickly look at a few possible curveball questions.

- Imagine you have the power to implement one global change in healthcare policy. What would it be and why?

- Describe a time when you had to make a decision without all the necessary information. How did you handle it?

- If you could have a conversation with any historical medical figure, who would it be and what would you discuss?

- How would you handle a situation where a patient's demands conflict with your own ethical beliefs?

- Suppose technology has advanced to the point where AI can perform most tasks of a PA. How do you envision your role evolving?

- Imagine you've discovered a way to completely eradicate one disease. Which one do you choose, and why?

- If you were given the resources to conduct any medical research study without limitation, what would be the focus of your study?

- How would you deal with a colleague who is competent in their work but consistently rude to patients and staff?

- You find yourself on a desert island with three medications at your disposal. Which ones would you choose and why?

- During a routine check-up, you notice signs of abuse on a patient. They plead with you not to report it. How do you proceed?

Absolutely, these questions are crafted to stretch your thinking well past the usual interview fare. They're your chance to really strut your stuff when it comes to nifty problem solving, ethical pondering, and laying bare what drives you in this world of medicine. No need to pen an essay for each one—but hey, give them some good noodle time before the big day. Scribble a few thoughts if that helps spark the ole brain engine. It's like a pre-interview workout for your gray matter!

Wrapping Up

To wrap up this chapter, we've explored some of the curveball questions, potential quizzes, and the occasional writing samples you might encounter during your interview. While my personal experience varied—with some interviews featuring none of these elements and others presenting them in full force—I was always ready to tackle whatever came my way. I've shared these insights so that you, too, can step into your interviews with confidence.

Remember, being prepared is half the battle won. Now, let's tie up all that we've learned and close out the interview process with finesse, ensuring you come across as the consummate professional you're destined to be.

Chapter 9
Ending the Interview and the Art of Follow-Up

Congratulations! You've made it through the interview. But hold on just a minute—there's a nuanced art to properly concluding your interview and effectively following up. It's crucial to come prepared with questions for your interviewers. Typically, at the end of the interview they will turn the tables and ask if you have any questions. And you should have some. I've compiled a list of potential questions that you can pose to your interviewers. What worked well for me was not just asking a question but having a strategic follow-up question ready—preferably one that allows me to weave in my own strengths. Here's an example of how it might play out:

Interviewer: "Do you have any questions for us?"

You: "Yes, I have a few questions. To start, what would you say is the most important quality for a student to be successful in your program?"

Interviewer: "I believe the key is a student's ability to steer clear of distractions, remain focused, and commit to the intensity of the program."

You: "That aligns perfectly with my approach. I've organized my life to embrace this upcoming chapter fully. I've saved up, so I don't plan on working. I'll be living at home, where I can count on a quiet environment and my family's support. Plus, my fiancée is enrolled in an ultrasound program, so we're in sync about education being our top priority."

Notice how in this example I demonstrated that my personal circumstances and mindset are specifically designed to align with the demands of the program. This tactic underscores my commitment and suitability, potentially making a memorable impact on the interviewer. I advise that you do more than just come up with questions; prepare thoughtful follow-up responses as well. These should reinforce your candidacy and show that you're not only interested in the program but also primed to thrive in it.

Here some potential questions to ask your interviewers:

- Could you elaborate on the program's structure and the courses offered?

- Can you provide details about the clinical rotation schedule and the opportunities available?

- How is clinical experience integrated with classroom learning during the first year?

- What support services are available to students for academic and clinical success?

- Could you describe the mentorship opportunities within the program? Are there faculty or peer mentors for students?

- How do students typically fare on the PANCE, and what preparatory resources does the program provide?

- In what ways does the program encourage interprofessional collaboration and learning?

- Are there opportunities for students to participate in research or community outreach projects?

- How does the program use student feedback to improve the curriculum and clinical experiences continuously?

- Can you share examples of recent graduates' employment outcomes, or how the program assists with job placement?

- What is the program's philosophy on patient care, and how does this philosophy manifest in the training process?

- How does the program prepare students for the changing landscape of the PA profession and future healthcare developments?

These questions are designed to show that you're considering how the program will fit your educational needs and career goals, while also demonstrating your proactive approach to becoming a well-rounded PA.

Follow Up to Stand Out

As we're winding down the interview, let's add those final professional touches. It's always a good idea to ask for a business card or email contact from your interviewers. Why? Well, it gives you the chance to shoot them a thank you email 24 hours later, showing your appreciation for the opportunity.

Now, not everyone might expect this, but in my book, it's a small gesture that sets you apart as a true professional. It shows you value their time and the opportunity they've given you, and that's something that definitely leaves a positive impression.

So, here's a little template to get you started:

Dear Jennifer,

I wanted to thank you for the interview yesterday and for sharing so much about Summit View's PA program.

I was impressed by the many clinical affiliations Summit View's program has in the Long Island and NY Metro area. It was reassuring to hear you and your team emphasize the importance of supporting students to ensure their success. My interest in Summit View's PA program was already strong, but meeting with you and your team reinforced my desire to be part of your program. It's clear that you and the Summit View's staff are dedicated to producing top-notch PAs and providing excellent training.

I look forward to hearing back from Summit View once decisions are made. Thank you for your time and consideration. Please feel free to reach out if you have any further questions.

Thanks again,

Frank

See, my email is straight forward and to the point. It mentions key points from our conversation, and reaffirms my interest in the program. Even if they haven't made their final decisions yet, you will definitely make a strong impression by reaching out like this. Your name will surely stick in their minds for all the right reasons!

Chapter 10
Closing Remarks and Conclusion

As we turn the final page of this guide, I hope you feel equipped and ready. We've covered substantial ground—from choosing the right attire to maintaining composure on the day of the interview. We've tackled those challenging questions head-on and mapped out strategies to address them, not to mention honing the art of a thoughtful follow-up. This book is designed to be a resource you can return to time and again. Whenever you need a refresher, simply turn to the relevant chapter or section—no need to comb through from cover to cover each time.

The profession of physician assistant is, I believe, one of the most rewarding careers one can pursue. It has brought me immense joy and satisfaction, a comfortable lifestyle, and a place of respect within my community. You've made a commendable choice in aspiring to this path. As you embark on this journey toward securing a place in your chosen PA program and eventually stepping into the role of a PA, I trust you'll find the same profound gratification that I have found.

I wish you all the best as you move forward. May your path be smooth and lead you to a fulfilling career. I look forward to the day when you, too, are a colleague in this noble field. Godspeed on your journey.

Bonus Section
Question Bank

You've made it to the question bank section of this guide—well done! This part is the cherry on top, specially crafted to give you that extra edge for acing your PA school interview. While the question bank offers a comprehensive look at potential interview questions, consider this section your strategic playbook for turning preparation into a compelling performance.

Think of this question bank as a gold mine of scenarios that captures the essence of a PA's multifaceted role. It isn't exhaustive, but serves as a powerful tool to explore a spectrum of situations, from deeply empathetic encounters to the intricacies of ethical decision making. When you rehearse with your support system—be it friends, family, or mentors—try to recreate the interview atmosphere. This not only builds comfort and confidence, but also sharpens your ability to think and articulate under pressure.

Applying the STARR method to your practice can turn your responses from good to great, infusing them with a narrative quality that interviewers find engaging and insightful. It's all about storytelling with a professional twist—painting a picture of your experiences that clearly illustrates your skills and growth. Dive into your personal history to find those golden moments that align with the themes of the question bank. Each question is an invitation to showcase how you stand out, not just in your knowledge and experience, but in your capacity for reflection and growth. So, take these tips, weave them into your practice, and step into your PA school interview ready to shine!

Empathy and Patient Care

- How would you describe the role of empathy in patient care?

- How would you handle a situation where you felt a patient's request was not in their best health interest?

- What is your approach to building trust with a new patient?

- How do you balance compassion and professional detachment in patient care?

- Describe how you would respond to a patient who is upset or angry.

- Describe how you would manage a long-term patient relationship.

Healthcare Knowledge and Passion

- Can you discuss a healthcare topic you are passionate about, and how you stay informed?

- How do you plan to keep your medical knowledge up to date after graduation?

- Can you talk about an innovative idea you have for the PA profession?

- What are your thoughts on the importance of cultural competency in healthcare?

- How do you assess the credibility of a new research study or medical information?

Contributions to the PA Profession

- How do you plan to contribute to the PA profession outside of clinical practice?

- What do you believe is the biggest misconception about PAs, and how would you address it?

Adaptability and Change Management

- Tell me about a time when you had to adapt to a significant change in your academic or professional life.

- Describe a situation where you had to quickly learn something new to help a patient.

Ethics and Professional Responsibility

- Describe a situation where you had to balance your personal beliefs with professional responsibilities.

- How would you handle a situation where you made a mistake with a patient's treatment?

- How would you deal with a situation involving an ethical dilemma with a patient?

Teamwork and Conflict Resolution

- Describe your understanding of the interprofessional healthcare team and the PA's role within it.

- Can you provide an example of how you've handled conflict in a team setting?

- Describe a time when you took the initiative in a clinical or educational setting.

- How would you react if a treatment you suggested was not supported by your supervising physician?

- Can you talk about a time when you disagreed with a policy or procedure and how you handled it?

Personal Development and Self-Care

- What strategies do you use to maintain your mental health during stressful periods?

- Describe how you stay motivated during challenging times in your studies or work.

- Can you discuss the importance of self-care in the PA profession?

- How do you plan to balance the demands of a PA career with your personal life?

Innovation and Continuous Learning

- Discuss a time when you had to advocate for a cause or policy change.

- How do you approach setting goals for your professional development?

- How do you handle situations where you have limited resources to provide patient care?

- Discuss a professional challenge you anticipate facing as a PA and how you plan to overcome it.

- How do you prioritize tasks when everything seems urgent?

- What is your approach to dealing with uncertainty in a clinical setting?

Leadership and Initiative

- How would you address a situation where a patient is hesitant to follow medical advice due to misinformation?

- Can you discuss a time when you had to work under pressure?

- Describe a time when you went above and beyond for a patient or colleague.

- Can you give an example of a time when you received constructive feedback and how you applied it?

- Discuss a time when you had to make a decision without all the desired information.

- How would you handle a situation where you need to deliver difficult news to a patient?

- How do you approach making decisions in a high-stakes environment?

- Describe a situation where you had to prioritize patient safety over efficiency.

- How would you address a situation where you suspect a patient is not being truthful?

- Can you discuss a time when you had to advocate for patient education?

- Describe how you would handle a situation where a patient's wishes conflict with their family's wishes.

- What is your approach to ensuring that you are culturally sensitive to all patients?

- How do you handle situations where you have to work with limited patient information?

- Describe a scenario where you had to utilize your problem-solving skills in patient care.

- Can you discuss a time when you had to take a leadership role unexpectedly in a clinical setting?

Made in the USA
Las Vegas, NV
06 September 2024